W9-DIT-229

20 FUN FACTS ABOUT THE DIGESTIVE SYSTEM

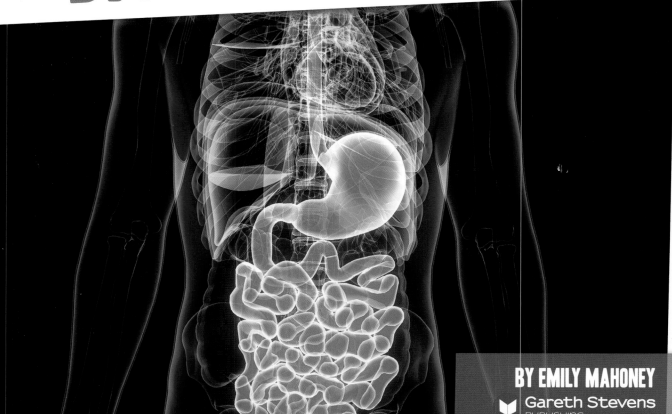

BY EMILY MAHONEY

Gareth Stevens
PUBLISHING

Please visit our website, www.garethstevens.com. For a free color catalog of all our high-quality books, call toll free 1-800-542-2595 or fax 1-877-542-2596.

Library of Congress Cataloging-in-Publication Data

Names: Mahoney, Emily Jankowski, author.
Title: 20 fun facts about the digestive system / Emily Mahoney.
Description: New York : Gareth Stevens Publishing, [2019] | Series: Fun fact file: body systems | Includes index.
Identifiers: LCCN 2018022956| ISBN 9781538229224 (library bound) | ISBN 9781538232743 (pbk.) | ISBN 9781538232750 (6 pack)
Subjects: LCSH: Digestion–Juvenile literature. | Gastrointestinal system–Physiology–Juvenile literature.
Classification: LCC QP145 .M32 2019 | DDC 612.3–dc23
LC record available at https://lccn.loc.gov/2018022956

First Edition

Published in 2019 by
Gareth Stevens Publishing
111 East 14th Street, Suite 349
New York, NY 10003

Copyright © 2019 Gareth Stevens Publishing

Designer: Sarah Liddell
Editor: Meta Manchester

Photo credits: Cover, p. 1 (main) Life science/Shutterstock.com; file folder used throughout David Smart/Shutterstock.com; binder clip used throughout luckyraccoon/Shutterstock.com; wood grain background used throughout ARENA Creative/Shutterstock.com; p. 5 La Gorda/Shutterstock.com; p. 6 Tom Wang/Shutterstock.com; p. 7 Irina Bg/Shutterstock.com; p. 8 Sergey Novikov/Shutterstock.com; pp. 9, 11 Designua/Shutterstock.com; pp. 10, 22 MDGRPHCS/Shutterstock.com; p. 12 Magic mine/Shutterstock.com; p. 13 decade3d - anatomy online/Shutterstock.com; p. 14 ilusmedical/Shutterstock.com; p. 15 solar22/Shutterstock.com; pp. 16, 25 sciencepics/Shutterstock.com; p. 17 igorwheeler/Shutterstock.com; p. 18 Nerthuz/Shutterstock.com; p. 19 nobeastsofierce/Shutterstock.com; p. 20 Treetree2016/Shutterstock.com; p. 21 bitt24/Shutterstock.com; p. 23 Aleksandr Andreev/Shutterstock.com; p. 24 Anatomy Insider/Shutterstock.com; p. 26 Alex Mit/Shutterstock.com; p. 27 ben bryant/Shutterstock.com; p. 29 karelnoppe/Shutterstock.com.

All rights reserved. No part of this book may be reproduced in any form without permission in writing from the publisher, except by a reviewer.

Printed in the United States of America

CPSIA compliance information: Batch #CW19GS: For further information contact Gareth Stevens, New York, New York at 1-800-542-2595.

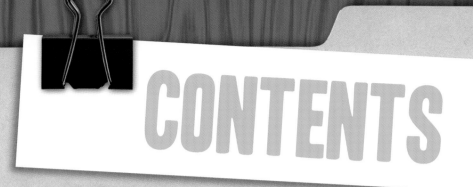

CONTENTS

Words in the glossary appear in **bold** type the first time they are used in the text.

DIGESTING THE FACTS

The digestive system is one of the most complex (and grossest!) systems in the human body. When you digest the food you eat, it's **converted** into energy that your body uses to think, work, and play.

The food you eat moves through the digestive system, starting in the mouth. When you swallow, food goes down the esophagus and into the stomach. From there, it travels through the small and large intestines, then out the anus. During the whole process, food is broken down into simpler matter the body can use.

THE DIGESTIVE SYSTEM

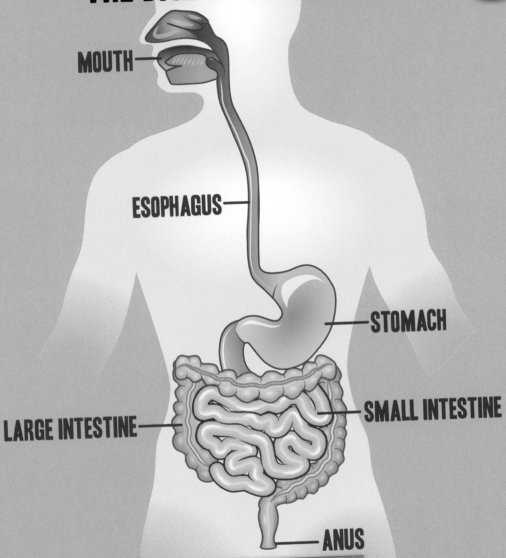

MOUTH

ESOPHAGUS

STOMACH

SMALL INTESTINE

LARGE INTESTINE

ANUS

The human digestive system has a lot of parts packed into a small space!

THE MIGHTY MOUTH

THE HARDEST MATERIAL IN YOUR BODY IS IN YOUR MOUTH.

Enamel is the material that makes up the outermost part of your teeth. It's very hard—even harder than your bones! It **protects** your teeth while you eat and drink. Chewing is the first step in digestion, so strong enamel is important!

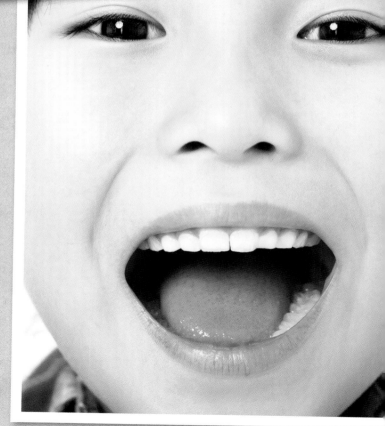

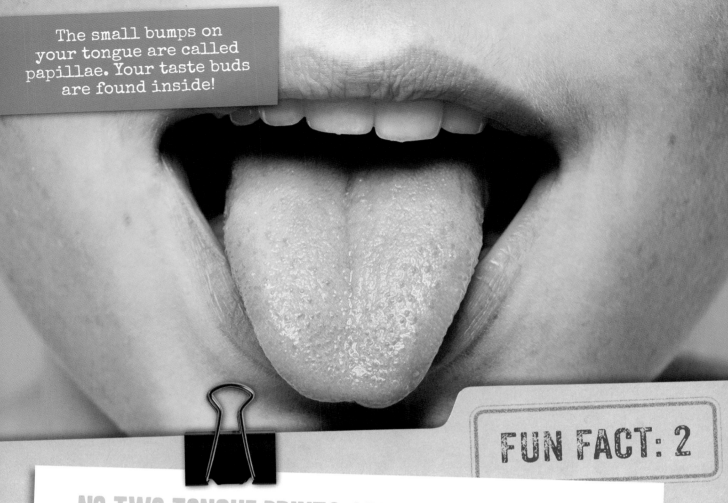

The small bumps on your tongue are called papillae. Your taste buds are found inside!

FUN FACT: 2

NO TWO TONGUE PRINTS ARE EXACTLY THE SAME!

It's not likely anyone will ask for your tongue print to figure out who you are, but your tongue is still important. It helps keep food between your teeth while you chew. It also helps you swallow.

7

THE EXCITING ESOPHAGUS

FUN FACT: 3

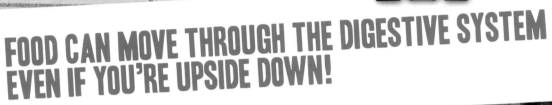

FOOD CAN MOVE THROUGH THE DIGESTIVE SYSTEM EVEN IF YOU'RE UPSIDE DOWN!

Wavelike muscle movement pushes food through the esophagus. This action of muscles contracting and **relaxing** is called peristalsis.

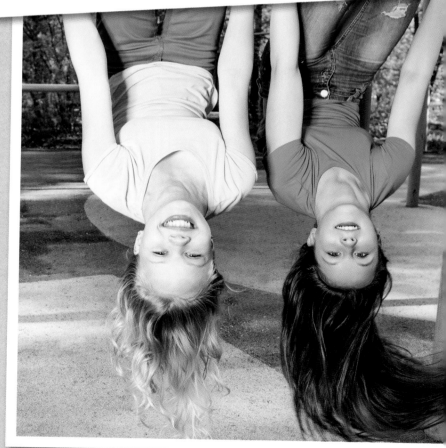

PERISTALSIS

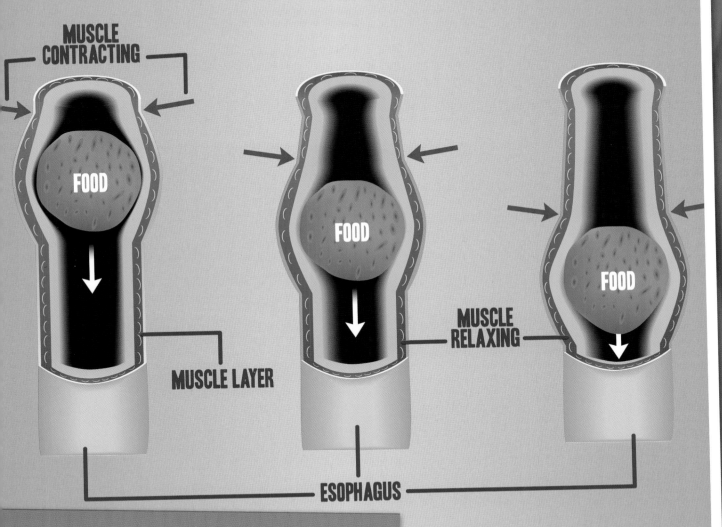

MUSCLE CONTRACTING

FOOD

FOOD

FOOD

MUSCLE LAYER

MUSCLE RELAXING

ESOPHAGUS

Muscles are the parts of the body that allow movement. The muscles in the esophagus work no matter what position you're in!

IT TAKES LESS THAN 10 SECONDS FOR FOOD TO MOVE THROUGH THE ESOPHAGUS TO THE STOMACH.

Peristalsis moves food through the esophagus surprisingly quickly. You can sometimes feel the food moving down your esophagus if you swallow something too large or without chewing it enough.

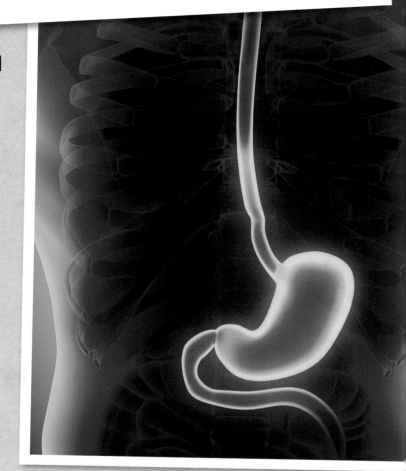

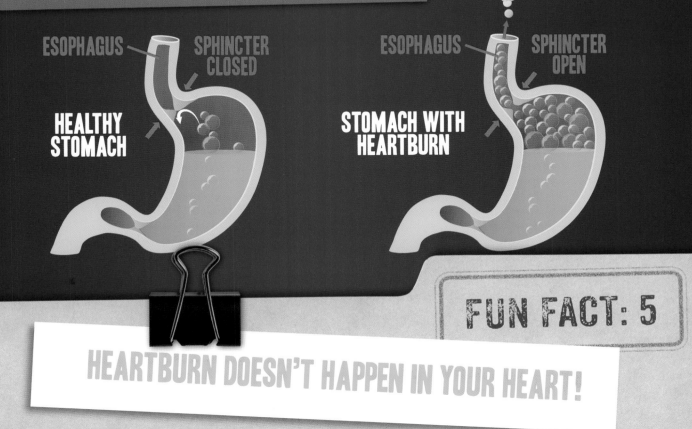

The lower esophageal sphincter is the muscle between the esophagus and stomach.

ESOPHAGUS   SPHINCTER CLOSED

HEALTHY STOMACH

ESOPHAGUS   SPHINCTER OPEN

STOMACH WITH HEARTBURN

FUN FACT: 5

HEARTBURN DOESN'T HAPPEN IN YOUR HEART!

Heartburn occurs when **acid** from the stomach comes back up into the esophagus, causing a burning feeling. This can happen if the muscle between the stomach and esophagus stays relaxed or becomes weak.

STOMACH STUFF

YOUR STOMACH ISN'T WHERE YOU THINK IT IS!

If you have a tummy ache, you might hold your belly, down near your belly button. But your stomach is actually higher up on the left side of your body, closer to your ribs!

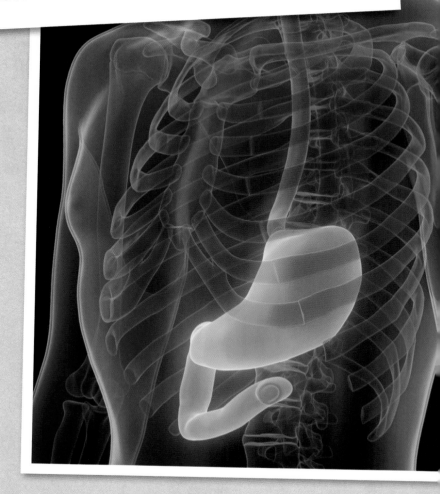

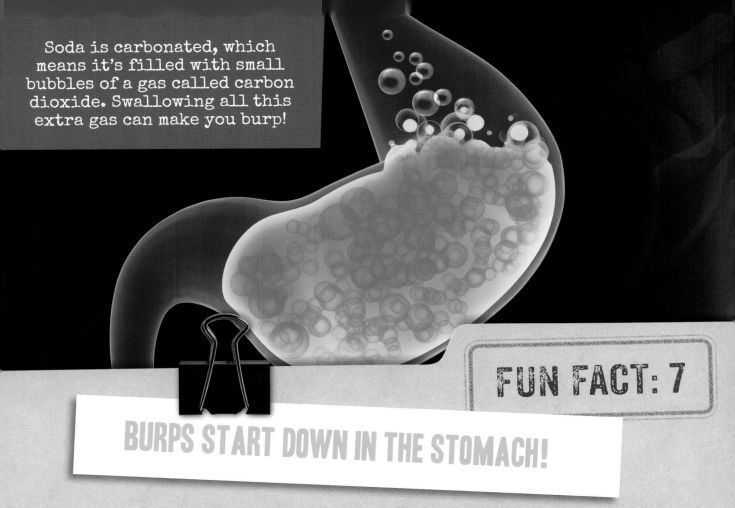

Soda is carbonated, which means it's filled with small bubbles of a gas called carbon dioxide. Swallowing all this extra gas can make you burp!

BURPS START DOWN IN THE STOMACH!

When you eat, you swallow food and air. This air leaves your body by traveling out of the stomach, up the esophagus, and out the mouth as a loud burp. If the air stays trapped in your stomach, it can give you a tummy ache. This is why babies cry if they aren't burped after they eat.

STOMACH ACID IS STRONG ENOUGH TO DESTROY YOUR ORGANS.

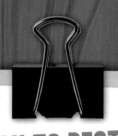

But don't worry! Your stomach produces new mucus every 2 weeks. Mucus is a thick liquid that protects the stomach from the acid needed to digest food.

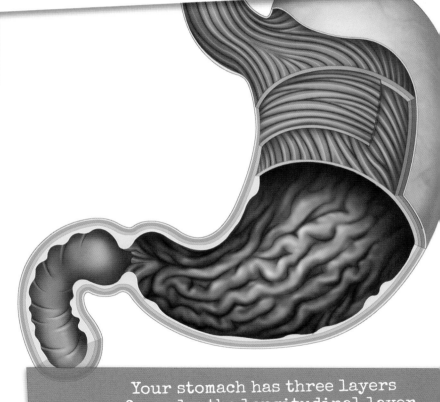

Your stomach has three layers of muscle: the longitudinal layer on the outside, the circular layer in the middle, and the oblique layer on the inside.

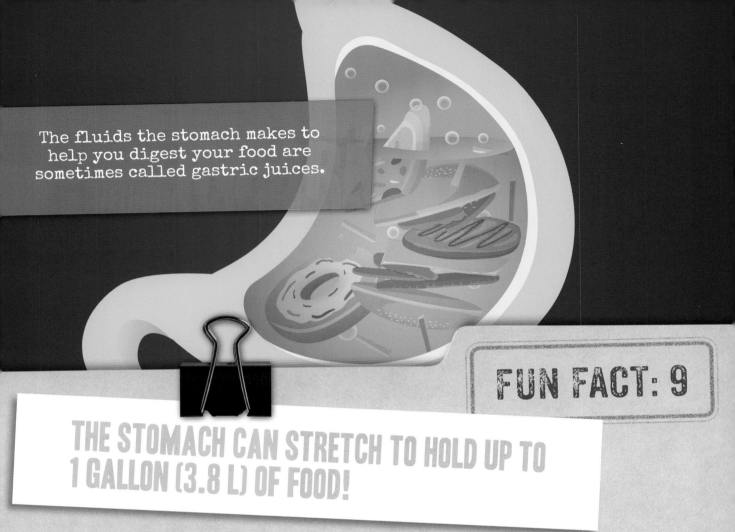

The fluids the stomach makes to help you digest your food are sometimes called gastric juices.

FUN FACT: 9

THE STOMACH CAN STRETCH TO HOLD UP TO 1 GALLON (3.8 L) OF FOOD!

Eating smaller amounts of food is a good idea, though, because it's easier for the stomach to break it down. Partly digested food, called chyme, then moves into the small intestine.

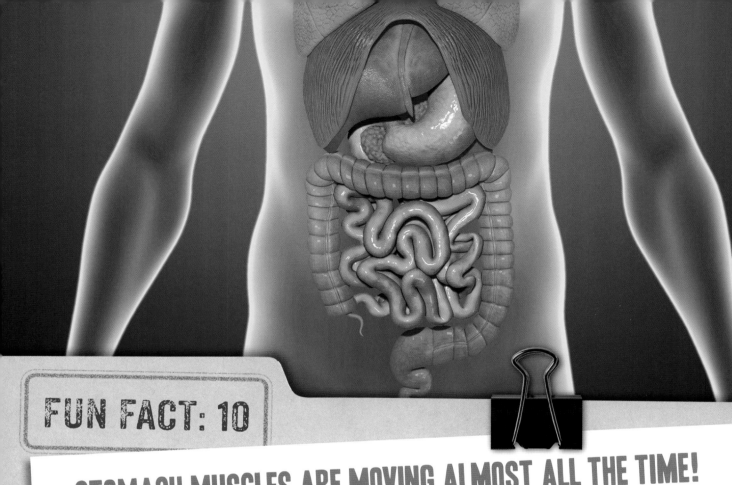

STOMACH MUSCLES ARE MOVING ALMOST ALL THE TIME!

They contract and relax to mix up food as it breaks down. When the food is ready, the muscles pump the chyme down toward the small intestine. The muscles even contract and relax when your stomach is empty, which makes your stomach rumble!

GUM DOESN'T ACTUALLY TAKE 7 YEARS TO DIGEST.

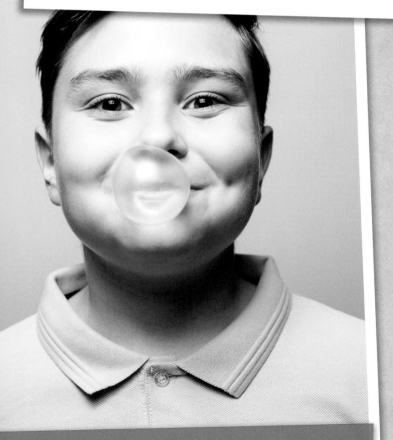

Swallowing one piece of gum won't harm you, but it's still better to throw it out when you're done chewing it.

One reason is because your body can't digest most of what gum is made of at all! A piece of gum will move through your digestive system mostly unchanged over the course of a few days until it leaves your body with other waste.

THE SMALL INTESTINE

FUN FACT: 12

AN ADULT'S SMALL INTESTINE IS ABOUT 22 FEET (6.7 M) LONG!

It's packed into your **abdomen** and absorbs, or takes in, **nutrients** from food. Even though it's long, it's only about 1 inch (2.5 cm) around.

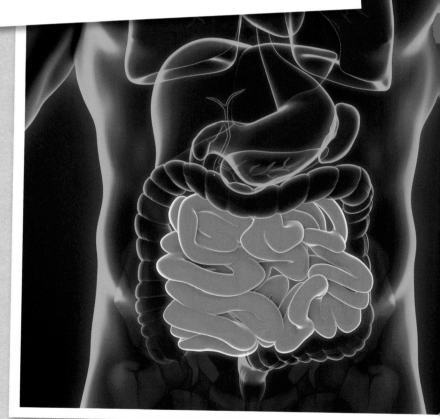

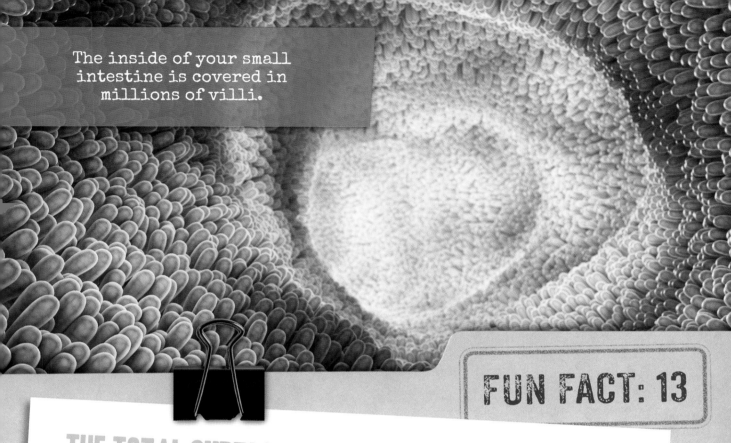

The inside of your small intestine is covered in millions of villi.

THE TOTAL SURFACE AREA OF THE SMALL INTESTINE IS ABOUT THE SAME SIZE AS A TENNIS COURT!

This is partly because of finger-like structures called villi that absorb, or take in, the nutrients from food. The villi increase the surface area of the small intestine, which allows more nutrients to be absorbed in a shorter time.

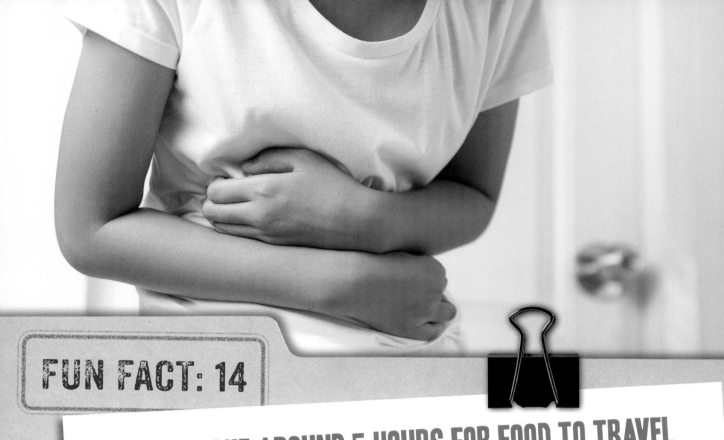

IT CAN TAKE AROUND 5 HOURS FOR FOOD TO TRAVEL THROUGH THE SMALL INTESTINE.

The whole time, muscles chop chyme up into very tiny pieces so the body can absorb nutrients. When you eat too much food at one time, these muscles might cramp up and make you feel uncomfortable.

YOUR BODY DOESN'T DIGEST FIBER, BUT YOU STILL NEED TO EAT IT.

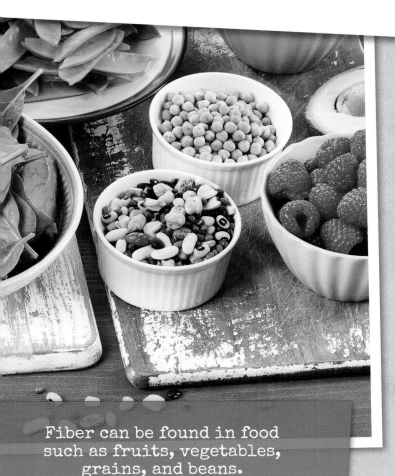

Fiber can be found in food such as fruits, vegetables, grains, and beans.

Fiber is an important part of a healthy **diet** because it helps you feel full and digest sugar slower. It also keeps food moving through the intestines, so it's good to eat if you're feeling blocked up.

FUN FACT: 16

YOU CAN LIVE WITHOUT YOUR LARGE INTESTINE.

The main job of your large intestine, also called the colon, is to keep you **hydrated** by removing water from the waste from the small intestine. If the colon becomes unhealthy, it can be removed.

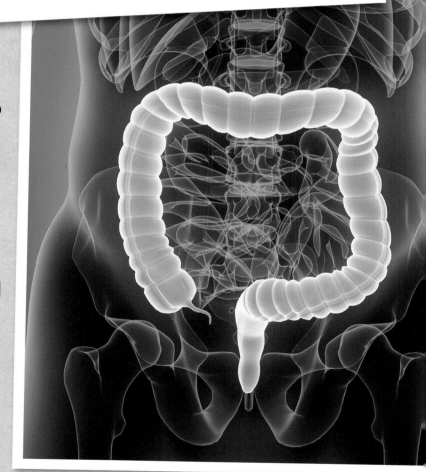

LENGTH OF THE DIGESTIVE SYSTEM

MOUTH ————

ESOPHAGUS ————

STOMACH ————

SMALL INTESTINE ————

LARGE INTESTINE ————

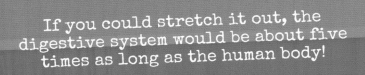

If you could stretch it out, the digestive system would be about five times as long as the human body!

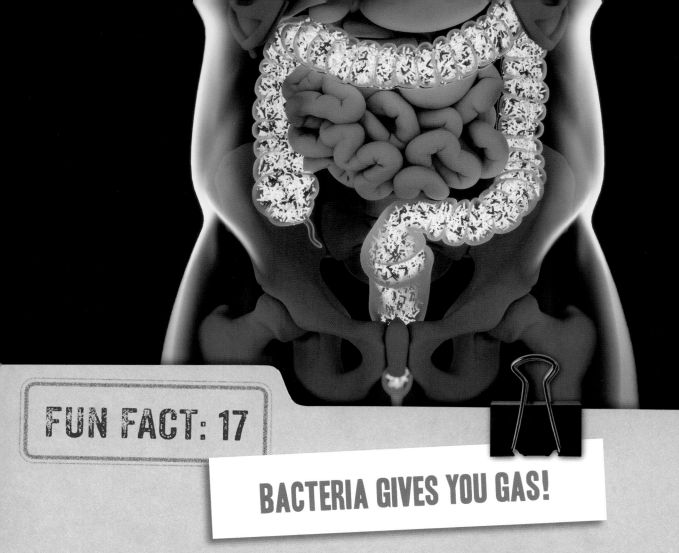

BACTERIA GIVES YOU GAS!

Have you ever loudly passed gas at a bad time?

Bacteria in the large intestine can cause waste to **ferment**,

producing gas. The only way for that gas to exit the body

is . . . well, you know!

THE LARGE INTESTINE IS SHORTER THAN THE SMALL INTESTINE.

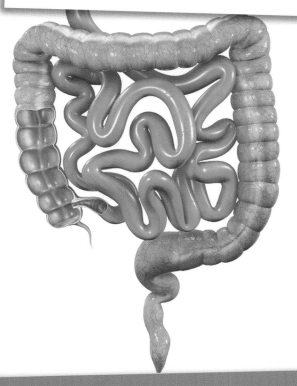

Though it's only about 5 feet (1.5 m) long, the large intestine can hold food for more than a day. During this time, it removes water from waste. What's left is called stool, or poop!

The large intestine may not be as long as the small intestine, but it's much wider. In fact, at about 3 inches (7.6 cm) around, it's about three times as wide!

THE END OF THE LINE

THE RECTUM IS THE LAST STOP BEFORE WASTE LEAVES THE BODY.

The end of the large intestine is called the rectum. The rectum connects the rest of the digestive system to the anus. There are **receptors** in the walls of the rectum that tell you when you need to use the bathroom.

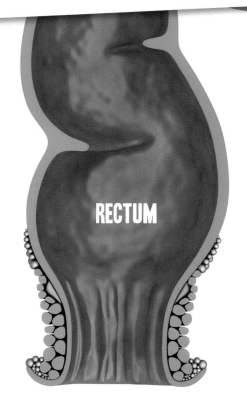

RECTUM

26

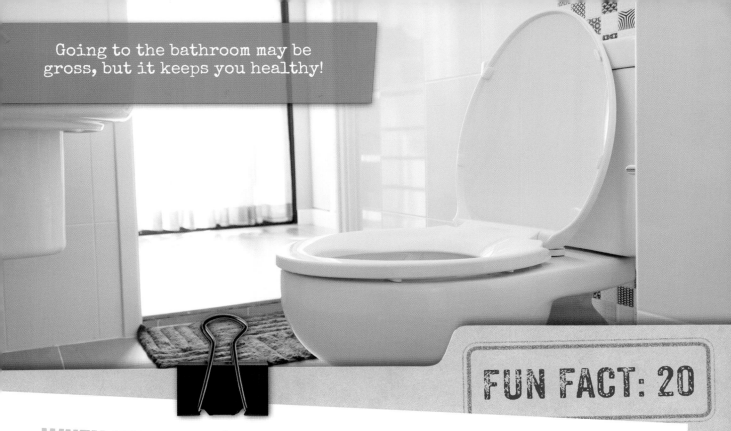

Going to the bathroom may be gross, but it keeps you healthy!

WHEN YOU POOP, YOU'RE ACTUALLY GETTING RID OF FOOD FROM DAYS AGO, NOT WHAT YOU ATE THAT DAY!

Food takes about 24 to 72 hours to pass through your digestive system. The amount of time changes based on what you eat, whether you're male or female, how active you are, and if you have certain health problems.

27

AN AMAZING JOURNEY

The foods you eat go on a long journey through the digestive system. They change a lot as they move from mouth to rectum. The digestive system helps give your body energy and get rid of waste.

The next time you eat lunch or grab a snack, you'll have a better idea of how your body gets nutrition and energy from your hamburger, spaghetti, or salad. Make sure to eat healthy foods. Your amazing digestive system will thank you for it!

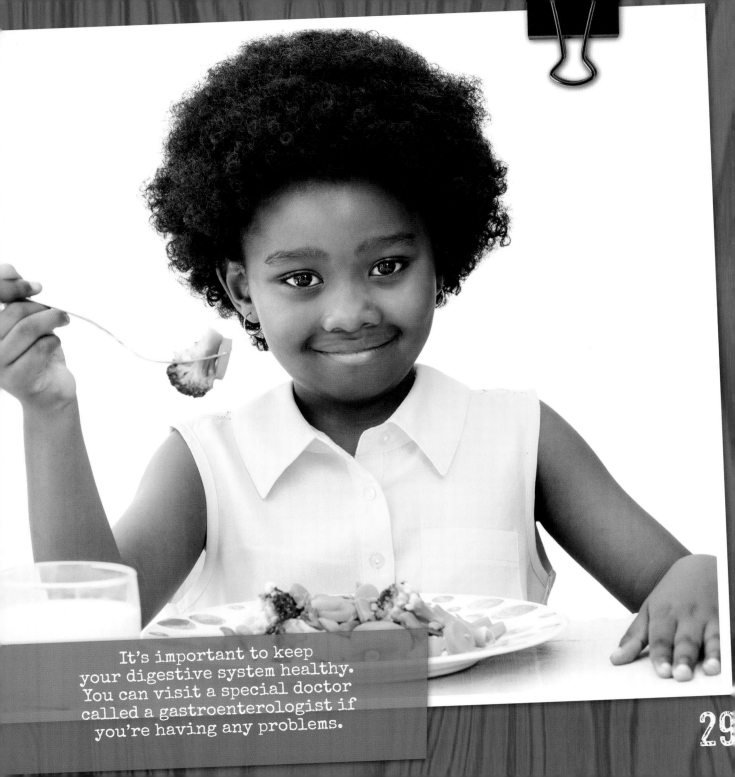

It's important to keep your digestive system healthy. You can visit a special doctor called a gastroenterologist if you're having any problems.

GLOSSARY

abdomen: the part of the body below the chest that contains the stomach and other organs

acid: a liquid that breaks down matter

convert: to cause to change form

diet: the food a person usually eats

ferment: to go through a chemical change that results in the production of alcohol

hydrated: having a healthy amount of water in the body

material: matter from which something is made

nutrient: something a living thing needs to grow and stay alive

organ: a part inside an animal's body

protect: to keep safe

receptor: a special body part that senses changes in light, temperature, or pressure and causes the body to react in a certain way

relax: to become less tense, tight, or stiff

surface area: the amount of area covered by the surface of something

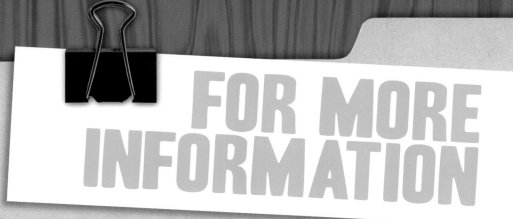

FOR MORE INFORMATION

BOOKS

Activity Book Zone for Kids. *The Stomach and More: Digestive System Coloring Book.* United Kingdom: Sabeels Publishing, 2016.

Co, Gomdori. *Survive! Inside the Human Body, Vol. 1: The Digestive System.* San Francisco, CA: No Starch Press, 2013

DK. *Human Body!* New York, NY: DK Publishing, 2017.

WEBSITES

Body Systems

www.dkfindout.com/us/human-body/your-amazing-body/body-systems/
Learn more about the digestive system and other body systems.

Follow Your Food

www.natgeokids.com/uk/discover/science/general-science/digestive-system/
National Geographic Kids presents a fun journey through the digestive system.

Your Digestive System

kidshealth.org/en/kids/digestive-system.html
Find great information about the digestive system here.

Publisher's note to educators and parents: Our editors have carefully reviewed these websites to ensure that they are suitable for students. Many websites change frequently, however, and we cannot guarantee that a site's future contents will continue to meet our high standards of quality and educational value. Be advised that students should be closely supervised whenever they access the internet.

31

INDEX